MCQs FOR THE DRCOG

Dedicated to Sue, Carrie, Lisa, Richard, Ellie, Edward, Anna, Fiona and to the continuation of the Northern Ireland peace process

For Churchill Livingstone:

Commissioning Editor: Ellen Green
Project Editors: Sarah Keer-Keer & Jane Shanks
Project Controller: Nancy Arnott
Designer: Erik Bigland

MCQs for the DRCOG

Matthew Hoghton MB ChB MRCP(UK) DRCOG FPcert MRCGP

General Practitioner, Bristol

Patrick Hogston MB BS BSc LRCP FRCS MRCOG

Consultant Obstetrician and Gynaecologist,
St Mary's Hospital, Portsmouth
Clinical Teacher, University of Southampton

Foreword by
Gordon M. Stirrat MA MD FRCOG

Professor of Obstetrics and Gynaecology,
University of Bristol, Bristol

SECOND EDITION

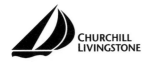

CHURCHILL
LIVINGSTONE

EDINBURGH LONDON NEW YORK PHILADELPHIA SYDNEY TORONTO 1999

CHURCHILL LIVINGSTONE
An imprint of Harcourt Brace and Company Limited

© Harcourt Brace and Company Limited 1999

⚓ is a registered trademark of Harcourt Brace and Company Limited

First edition 1991
Second edition 1999

ISBN 0443 062471

British Library Cataloguing in Publication Data
A catalogue record for this book is available from the British Library.

Library of Congress Cataloging in Publication Data
A catalog record for this book is available from the Library of Congress.

Note
Medical knowledge is constantly changing. As new information becomes available, changes in treatment, procedures, equipment and the use of drugs become necessary. The authors and the publishers have, as far as it is possible, taken care to ensure that the information given in this text is accurate and up-to-date. However, readers are strongly advised to confirm that the information, especially with regard to drug usage, complies with the latest legislation and standards of practice.

The
publisher's
policy is to use
**paper manufactured
from sustainable forests**

Printed in China

FOREWORD TO THE FIRST EDITION

If, as we are told, confession is good for the soul I should feel better after writing this foreword. The fact of the matter is that I dislike MCQs. No, let me be more accurate – I *detest* them. Why do I feel so strongly about this widely used form of assessment? My first reason is that the structure of the questions often requires definite decisions about variable and indefinite issues. Second, this form of examination was being introduced experimentally when I was a student and I do not think I passed any of them!

I suspect that my feelings towards MCQs are shared by a great many but there is no doubt that as a form of assessment MCQs are here to stay and we have to accommodate to them. That is why this excellent book by Matthew Hoghton and Patrick Hogston is so welcome for candidates for the DRCOG.

Having accepted the invitation to write this foreword I felt that I had to put myself to the test. I therefore 'sat the exam'. You will be pleased to hear that I passed (although I did mark it myself). My mark must remain secret because I did not gain 90 let alone 100%! My errors fell into the following categories: (1) I didn't know and guessed (fatal!); (2) I thought I knew and was wrong (OK, so no-one's perfect!); (3) I misread the stem (stupid); and (4) I disagreed with the given answer (a professor's prerogative!).

Can I therefore reinforce the instructions given to you by the authors at the beginning of the book. The technique for MCQs is different, and can be practised and improved upon. Having answered the questions in this book once, review your marks and repeat the process until you begin to be satisfied with your performance (and then do it again). You will not only be more proficient at the technique but will have learned a great deal about the topics.

Let me therefore finally commend this book strongly to you as of great potential value for those sitting the DRCOG, I'm sorry I can't write any more – I have to take the exam again!

Gordon M. Stirrat

PREFACE TO SECOND EDITION

Reviewing and updating a book is similar to having to redecorate a room for a second time, i.e. it is often harder and you are never quite sure when the job is finished. Over the past seven years there have been new advances in medication and surgical techniques but what has surprised us is how much has not altered. The advice of the lecturer who tells you that 50% of what he is about to tell you will be incorrect in 10 years has yet to be proved. Clearly, one of the most important advances in medicine has been evidence-based medicine (EBM), which has sifted through research material to find useful and true information for doctors at the coalface.

In this second edition we have strengthened the answers with references and increased the number of questions by 20%. We hope that this book will help you pass your examination in the short-term and be part of your life long learning. If you want to comment, agree or disagree with our questions please contact us on od99@dial.pipex.com.

M.H.
P.H.

PREFACE TO FIRST EDITION

Since January 1990, the Diploma Examination of the Royal College of Obstetricians and Gynaecologists (DRCOG) has introduced Multiple Choice Questions into the written paper. Most candidates will have little opportunity to practise MCQ questions and hence the need for this book.

The aim of these practice examinations is to allow candidates to assess their knowledge under exam conditions. The answers are given at the end of each examination along with an explanation and further information where relevant. An index is included which will help the candidate to ensure he/she has covered the important topics. We have also provided a small list of recommended books.

M.H.
P.H.

ACKNOWLEDGEMENTS

We are grateful to Sarah Keer-Keer and Jane Shanks of Churchill Livingstone for supporting us in this endeavour. We are also grateful to the following contributors: Dr S. J. Armstrong MRCP, FRCR, Consultant Radiologist, Southmead Hospital, Bristol; Mr P. Curtis MRCOG, Consultant in Obstetrics and Gynaecology, Guildford Hospital, Surrey; and Miss S. Whitcroft MRCOG, Consultant in Obstetrics and Gynaecology, Guildford Hospital, Surrey.

CONTENTS

THE DRCOG: REGULATIONS, EXAMS AND CURRICULUM

DRCOG regulations

The DRCOG is an examination organised by the Royal College of Obstetricians and Gynaecologists. In order to enter the exam you should:

1. Have full registration with General Medical Council or by the Medical Council of Ireland.
2. Complete an application form from the Examination Secretary of the Royal College of Obstetricians and Gynaecologists, 27 Sussex Place, Regent's Park, London NW1 4RG, UK. Tel: +44 (0)171 772 6200, Fax: +44 (0)171 772 6359. The latest date for receiving such applications is 1st February for the April examination or 1st August for the October examination but these dates may vary.
3. Send the entry fee in sterling at the time of application. The current amount of the entry fee is £150. You must send a cheque made payable to 'The Royal College of Obstetricians and Gynaecologists'. You must not send cash.
4. Have finished a recognised combined appointment for 6 consecutive months. It is not essential to complete this training by the time of the examination. However, you will be required to provide a certificate confirming the completion of 6 months recognised training at the time of registration as a Diplomate of the College. In special circumstances part-time clinical training in recognised posts is permitted provided approval of the College is obtained in advance. These training posts must be held in the United Kingdom or Republic of Ireland.
5. Provide evidence of identification, which includes name and photograph, for inspection prior to commencement of the examination. Candidates failing to provide satisfactory evidence will not be allowed to attend the examination. When you are successful you are required to pay a registration fee and, at the same time, provide a certificate confirming the completion of 6 months recognised training before being granted the Diploma of the Royal College of Obstetricians and Gynaecologists. The amount of the current registration fee is available from the Examination Secretary.

Try and get it first time. You cannot take it more than 5 times!

The DRCOG exam

The examination is in two parts:

1. A multiple choice question (MCQ) paper lasting 2 hours examining areas of obstetrics, gynaecology and associated subjects. The paper consists of 60 five-part questions.
2. An objective structured clinical examination (OSCE). This part of the examination may cover obstetrics, gynaecology, neonatology, family planning or related subjects. There are 22 stations, each of 6 minutes, through which candidates rotate. Two of the stations are rest stations, whilst at each of the other stations a task will be performed. These tasks may be a test of factual knowledge, problem solving, diagnosis, investigation and treatment or communication skills.

The DRCOG curriculum

The Royal College of Obstetrics publishes the following guidelines. You should:

- appreciate the preventive role, and understand the significance of all routine procedures used in modern antenatal care.
- have an understanding of the epidemiology of maternal and pernatal morbitity and mortality as well as ethnic variations.
- be able to discuss the management of complications and life-threatening emergencies in early pregnancy.
- appreciate when those pregnant women initially suitable for shared care or full care by the general practitioner require referral for specialist opinion or care.
- understand the principles for pre-pregnancy evaluation and counselling of women faced with possible or real problems of fetal malformation.
- know the methods by which congenital malformation of the fetus may be detected.
- be aware of the methods of, and provision for, education in pregnancy, childbirth and the care of the newborn.
- understand the importance of social and emotional factors in pregnancy and childbirth.
- be able to understand and appreciate the risks of all types of antenatal and intrapartum infection for the mother, fetus and newborn infant.
- understand the role of the general practitioner, the midwife and that of the different members of the health care team in care of pregnant women.
- understand the management of common conditions for which pregnant women are admitted to hospital, e.g. premature labour, pre-eclampsia, multiple pregnancy, fetal growth retardation, antepartum haemorrhage and maternal diseases.
- be able to recognise the symptoms and signs of the onset of labour.
- understand the principles, mechanisms and methods of management of normal and abnormal labour.

- understand the principles and methods which are used for the relief of pain in labour.
- understand the importance of accurate and detailed records in all aspects of obstetric care and recognise the value of such records in clinical audit.
- be able to carry out and discuss the routine examination of a newborn infant.
- understand and discuss the normal development of the newborn infant.
- recognise common diseases arising in the newborn infant.
- recognise congenital abnormalities in the newborn infant.
- understand how breast feeding is established and maintained.
- recognise and treat all sources of infection in the puerperium.
- recognise and understand the management of physical and psychological problems of the mother in the postnatal period, e.g. puerperal depression.
- understand the normal involutional processes in the postpartum period.
- understand the indications for maternal immunisation with anti-D and rubella vaccine and the importance of confirming their efficacy.

With regard to **intranatal care**, you should:

- understand the indications for the induction of labour.
- understand the physiology of uterine activity and the use of oxytocic drugs to augment uterine action.
- know the principles and practice of continuous fetal heart rate monitoring and acid–base studies.
- recognise and discuss the abnormalities that may occur in labour, e.g. fetal distress, haemorrhage, delay in labour, abnormal presentation, etc.
- be able to:

  (a) induce labour where appropriate.
  (b) provide obstetric analgesia and local anaesthesia, including pudendal block.
  (c) carry out a low forceps delivery and repair of the perineum.
  (d) resuscitate a shocked mother.
  (e) resuscitate a newborn baby.

- understand the management of other abnormalities of labour, e.g. breech, twins, shoulder distocia.
- be able to manage the third stage of labour including the management of postpartum haemorrhage and retained placenta.
- be able to discuss the management of episiotomies and lacerations.
- be aware of special arrangements needed for home confinments.
- be able to communicate with women in labour so that they understand the procedures proposed for their own safety and that of their babies.

With regard to **gynaecology** and **genito-urinary medicine**, you should:

* understand the role of the general practitioner in health education and preventive measures with regard to gynaecological diseases.
* be able to take a gynaecological history, carry out a full and appropriate examination and conduct relevant investigations on patients of all ages.
* understand the physical disorders due to congenital abnormalities of the female genital tract.
* understand the principles involved in counselling patients with psycho-sexual problems.
* be able to advise, investigate and manage patients complaining of infertility.
* be able to manage all types of abortions in general practice including diagnosis, emergency treatment and after-care.
* understand the management of common menstrual disorders and the steps required to diagnose benign lesions of the genital tract and the principles regarding their management.
* know the steps required for the detection of pre-malignant lesion of the cervix, the diagnosis of invasive neoplasia of the genital tract, and the general practitioner's role in the management of terminal cancer.
* understand the physiology and management of the menopause.
* understand the diagnosis and management of urinary tract disorders and of genital prolapse.
* understand the diagnosis and management of patients suffering from vaginal discharges, infections of the genital tract and common vulval lesions.
* understand sexually transmitted diseases and their treatment and control.

With regard to **family planning**, it is expected that you will have the same theoretical knowledge that is required by doctors who wish to take the Diploma of the Faculty of Family Planning and Reproduction Health Care of the RCOG, namely knowledge of:

* acceptability of contraception.
* choice of method and discussion of risks and benefits.
* all available contraceptive methods; necessary technical skills and management of associated complications including resuscitation.
* male and female sterilisation.
* abortion; counselling, legal aspects, techniques.
* sexually transmitted diseases.
* family planning services; organisation and administration (community, general practice, domiciliary and hospital).
* well woman care.

However, the College issues a caveat that it can discuss other topics that are relevant to general practice!

INSTRUCTIONS FOR THE MCQ PAPER IN OBSTETRICS AND GYNAECOLOGY FOR DRCOG

The DRCOG paper consists of 60 five-part multiple choice questions. The time allowed for completion of the MCQ examination is 2 hours. The answer sheet is marked by computer and must be completed in HB pencil only. Each lozenge of the answer sheet should be filled with a bold dark line; the compute cannot read a faint line. A rubber is provided.

Each question consists of an initial statement followed by five items identified by the letters a, b, c, d and e. The answer sheet contains a row of five boxes for each question labelled accordingly. In each box there are three lozenges labelled T for true, F for false and DK for don't know. If you know a particular item of a question to be true or false, black out either the true (T) or the false (F) lozenge. If you do not know the answer you must black out the don't know (DK) lozenge.

Specimen question and answers

During breast feeding:

a Mastitis may be resolved by continued breast feeding
b Superficial mastitis should be treated with antibiotics
c Twins will require supplementary bottle feeding
d Lactating women should drink extra fluids
e Demand feeding produces obese babies

Answers **a** and **b** are TRUE, **c**, **d** and **e** are FALSE
Your answer sheet to this question would look like this when correctly filled in:

A	B	C	D	E
T ●	T ●	T ○	T ○	T ○
F ○	F ○	F ●	F ●	F ●
DK ○	DK ○	DK ○	DK ○	DK ○

T means TRUE, F means FALSE, DK means DON'T KNOW

If you know the answer to **a**, **b**, **c** and **d** but do not know the answer to **e** then your answer sheet will be completed as follows:

T ⬬	T ⬬	T ◯	T ◯	T ◯
F ◯	F ◯	F ⬬	F ⬬	F ◯
DK ◯	DK ◯	DK ◯	DK ◯	DK ⬬

Each item correctly answered (i.e. a true statement indicated as true or a false statement indicated as false) is awarded one mark (+1). For each incorrect answer, one mark is deducted (–1). For those items marked don't know, no marks are awarded or deducted (0).

The completed question book will be collected at the end of the time allowed for the MCQ examination. The essay paper will then be issued. It is not possible to leave the examination hall between completion of the MCQ paper and the start of the essay paper.

GENERAL ADVICE FOR TAKING MCQ EXAMINATIONS

Preparation for taking examinations

1. Do plenty of MCQs.
2. Talk about Obstetrics and Gynaecology with your colleagues.
3. Ask for teaching from senior colleagues and attend lectures at every opportunity. Try to get involved in the discussions.
4. Practise techniques, e.g. essay plans, vivas.
5. Try to take regular exercise between periods of study.
6. Avoid too many stimulants, especially coffee (take up decaffeinated!).
7. Go to bed at a regular time.
8. Plan your available time to cover the subject matter, rather than spending too much time on detail.

Answering MCQs

1. Read the instructions carefully.
2. Fill in your name and candidate number.
3. Plan your time.
4. Allow at least 15 minutes for transcribing your answers on to the answer sheet.
5. You are unlikely to know definitely all the answers. If you have no knowledge about a particular subject, do not guess, but if you feel that you are more than 50% certain of the answer you should probably attempt it.
6. Mark your responses in the appropriate box.

Interpretation of terms

Maybe	– unlikely to be false
Always	– likely to be false
Usually	– over 60% occurrence
Characteristic	– if absent, the diagnosis is unlikely
Rarely	– less than 10%
Majority	– greater than 50%
Can occur	– if it has occurred once, it can occur again

After the examination

1. Remember that an exam is only an exam; failing it is not the end of the world. Many excellent senior doctors have retaken postgraduate exams.
2. Go and relax. Avoid post-mortems, especially with people anxious to discuss how well they did. Also avoid having to support and reassure others.
3. Don't belittle yourself.
4. Apart from pride, all you lose is money.
5. Look after your loved ones, remember they are taking the exam with you.

PAPER A
QUESTIONS

A1 **Blood pressure in pregnancy:**
  A Rises gradually from the first trimester until delivery
  B Should be measured using a large cuff if the upper arm circumference is greater than 35 cm
  C Will be artificially lowered if taken with the patient lying
  D Will show at least one reading of 140/90 mmHg in 20% of women
  E Phase V of Korotkoff's sound is used in the measurement of diastolic pressure

A2 **Pre-eclampsia:**
  A Is commoner in women with a previous miscarriage
  B May present with abdominal pain and vomiting
  C Is more common in smokers than in non-smokers
  D Is a common cause of symmetrical intra-uterine growth retardation
  E Can be treated with diuretics in early cases

A3 **The following conditions can be diagnosed by high resolution ultrasound at 20 weeks of pregnancy:**
  A Holoprosencephaly
  B Gastroschisis
  C Cystic fibrosis
  D Urethral valves
  E Hypoplastic left heart

A4 **A pregnant woman with asthma:**
  A Should not be treated with aminophylline
  B Can be safely treated with steroids
  C Is more vulnerable to 'status asthmaticus' in labour
  D Has at least twice the chance of having a child who will develop asthma than does a non-asthmatic woman
  E Should avoid beta-sympathomimetic drugs

A5 **Thromboembolic disease in pregnancy:**
A Is a major cause of maternal death
B Should be treated with coumarins in the first trimester
C Venography and isotope lung scanning must not be used
D Preventative treatment with subcutaneous heparin has no risk to the mother
E Is commoner in women after Caesarean section

A6 **The following are compatible with a normal outcome of pregnancy:**
A Blood pressure at booking of 140/100 mmHg
B Weight gain throughout pregnancy of 2 kg
C Severe lower limb oedema
D Blood urea of 12 mmol/l
E Thalassaemia major

A7 **In pregnancy:**
A A haemoglobin of 11 g/dl is the lower limit of normal according to WHO guidelines
B A low serum iron with a low total iron binding capacity suggests iron deficiency
C The overall total iron requirement is approximately 1000 mg
D Iron absorption is increased
E The plasma volume rises by about 1200 ml

A8 **The following statements about the neonate are true:**
A An Apgar score of 3 at 5 minutes predicts a 50% chance of subsequent cerebral palsy
B Continuous electronic fetal heart rate monitoring in labour reduces the incidence of cerebral palsy
C Poor feeding and jaundice may be the only signs of neonatal septicaemia
D The commonest cause of death in the first year of life is the sudden infant death syndrome (SIDS)
E Ophthalmia neonatorum is a notifiable disease

A9 **The following conditions have an autosomal recessive mode of inheritance:**
A Achondroplasia
B Phenylketonuria
C Tuberous sclerosis
D Huntingdon's chorea
E Retinitis pigmentosa

A10 **The following are risk factors for shoulder dystocia:**
A Maternal weight of 110 kg
B Rotational forceps delivery
C Gestational diabetes
D 42 weeks gestation
E Oxytocin augmentation for primary dysfunctional labour

A11 **Which of the following increase the risk of a Caesarean section in a primigravida at 41 weeks gestation?:**
   A   Fresh meconium liquor seen in labour
   B   Induction of labour for prolonged rupture of the membranes
   C   Continuous electronic fetal monitoring
   D   Oxytocin augmentation for secondary arrest at 8 cm
   E   Artificial rupture of membranes as part of active management of labour

A12 **Primary postpartum haemorrhage (PPH):**
   A   Is reduced by active management of the third stage of labour
   B   Is usually caused by trauma to the genital tract
   C   Is less common in multiparous women
   D   Is more common in women who experienced it in previous pregnancies
   E   When the cause of maternal death is often due to delay in performing hysterectomy

A13 **Carcinoma of the cervix:**
   A   Kills more women than carcinoma of the ovary
   B   Is more common in social class V
   C   May be related to the sexual behaviour of the woman's partner
   D   Killed fewer women in 1997 than 1990 in the UK due to the national screening programme
   E   Can be present with a normal cervical smear

A14 **Ectopic pregnancy:**
   A   Has a higher incidence in women with copper intra-uterine contraceptive devices (IUCDs) than sexually active women not using contraception
   B   Is excluded by the presence of an intra-uterine gestational sac on ultrasound
   C   Reduces the chance of the woman having a live child
   D   Is excluded by a negative serum beta human chorionic gonadotrophin (hCG)
   E   Accounts for 20% of pregnancies occurring after failed sterilisation

A15 **The combined oral contraceptive pill:**
   A   Is relatively safe to continue up to the age of 40 in a woman who does not smoke
   B   Alters glucose tolerance
   C   Increases the incidence of vaginal candidiasis
   D   May be used as a means of postcoital contraception
   E   Increases the risk of ovarian cancer

A16 **Hormone replacement therapy (HRT) for postmenopausal women:**
  A   Has similar risks to the combined oral contraceptive pill
  B   Reduces the incidence of fractures of the vertebral bodies
  C   Should be given as oestrogen-only in women post hysterectomy
  D   May increase the risk of breast cancer
  E   May reduce mortality from cardiovascular disease

A17 **Intra-uterine contraceptive devices (IUCDs):**
  A   Should not be inserted immediately after menstruation, as the device will be expelled
  B   Should be removed at the menopause
  C   Can be used 4 days after unprotected intercourse to prevent implantation
  D   Should be removed if possible if pregnancy occurs
  E   Cause more pelvic infection in nulliparous women than in parous women

A18 **A woman who complains of menorrhagia:**
  A   May be losing a normal amount of blood per month
  B   Can be successfully treated with non-steroidal anti-inflammatory drugs
  C   Is unlikely to be under 40 years of age
  D   Will be helped by a dilatation and curettage (D&C) in most cases
  E   Should be referred, if she is over 40 years of age, to a gynaecologist

A19 **A couple complain of inability to conceive after 2 years of unprotected intercourse:**
  A   The cause is more likely to be in the female partner
  B   Ovulation can be confirmed by estimating the Day 21 progesterone
  C   Are more likely to be over 35 years of age
  D   If a spontaneous pregnancy ensues, the likelihood of its being ectopic is greater than in the general population
  E   The cause could be Salazopyrin therapy in the male partner

A20 **Endometriosis:**
  A   Is associated with low parity
  B   Is worsened by intra-uterine contraceptive devices (IUCDs)
  C   Is a rare cause of haematuria
  D   Can be treated with continuous use of the combined oral contraceptive pill
  E   If the ovaries are surgically removed at 35 years of age, oestrogen replacement should be given

A21 **Spontaneous abortion at 8 weeks:**
  A Is uncommon once a live fetus has been seen on ultrasound
  B Is often due to chromosomal abnormalities in the conceptus
  C Can be prevented by injections of human chorionic gonadatrophin (hCG)
  D Should be treated with anti-D in rhesus-negative women
  E May lead to acute pelvic inflammatory disease

A22 **At the climacteric:**
  A The sensation of hot flushes is due to stimulation of the temperature regulation centre
  B The incidence of fractures starts to increase
  C Plasma cholesterol and triglyceride levels fall
  D Oestrogen therapy by vaginal cream does not result in endometrial hyperplasia
  E Hormone replacement therapy (HRT) increases the risk of thromboembolism

A23 **Ovarian cancer:**
  A May present with dyspepsia
  B Is commoner in social class V
  C Usually presents as stage I or II disease
  D Kills more women than all other gynaecological cancers
  E Is more common in previous users of the combined oral contraceptive pill

A24 **Secondary amenorrhoea:**
  A Is more common in athletes and ballet dancers
  B Often follows cessation of the oral contraceptive pill for at least 6 months
  C May follow dilatation and curettage (D&C)
  D May lead to osteoporosis
  E Due to ovarian failure, will cause a low serum FSH/LH ratio

A25 **Pre-term delivery:**
  A The risk is increased by smoking
  B Is more likely after a previous first trimester termination
  C Is less likely in diabetic women
  D Can be prevented by cervical cerclage in most cases
  E Occurs in approximately 15% of women admitted with painful contractions before 37 weeks

A26 **Therapy with beta-sympathomimetic drugs to treat pre-term labour:**
  A Improves the outcome for the baby
  B The drugs cross the placenta
  C Can cause fatal pulmonary oedema
  D Is contraindicated in asthmatics
  E Can cause hyperglycaemic ketoacidosis

A27 **Antenatal care should include:**
A Serial vaginal examination when there is a previous history of termination of pregnancy
B Testing for hepatitis B in women from Vietnam
C Haemoglobin electrophoresis in women from Pakistan
D Routine use of kick charts to prevent intra-uterine death
E Iron and folic acid supplements given to women with twins

A28 **Human immunodeficiency virus (HIV) infection:**
A Is associated with an increased risk of pre-term delivery
B Causes characteristic fetal abnormalities
C Can be transmitted in the breast milk
D Can cause maternal meningitis
E Is associated with squamous cell carcinoma of the rectum

A29 **The following are more common in the male child:**
A Talipes equinovarus
B Congenital dislocation of the hip
C Pyloric stenosis
D Isolated cleft palate
E Hirchsprung's disease

A30 **Physiological neonatal jaundice:**
A May occur on the first day after birth
B Will require phototherapy if the bilirubin rises to 200 μmol/l
C Will cause a positive Coombs' test
D Is better treated by bottle-feeding
E Is more common in pre-term babies

A31 **The pre-menstrual syndrome (PMS):**
A Is relieved by hysterectomy
B Is relieved by a sympathetic doctor
C Can be treated with spironolactone
D Lasts throughout the menstrual cycle
E Occurs while on the oral contraceptive pill

A32 **Depoprovera (medroxyprogesterone acetate):**
A Eventually causes amenorrhoea
B Cannot be given to women with sickle cell anaemia
C Is as effective as the combined oral contraceptive pill
D Can be given to lactating women
E Causes weight gain

A33 **The following may be diagnosed by chorionic villus biopsy:**
A Alpha thalassaemia
B Cystic fibrosis
C Haemophilia
D Edward's syndrome (trisomy 18)
E Fragile X syndrome

A34 **A woman with a raised serum alpha fetoprotein (AFP) at 16 weeks:**
- **A** Has a 50% chance of carrying a fetus with spina bifida
- **B** Is more significant if the woman is an insulin-dependent diabetic
- **C** Has an increased risk of a child with Down's syndrome
- **D** Should have a detailed ultrasound
- **E** May have an intra-uterine death

A35 **Breech presentation:**
- **A** Occurs in 2% of all labours at term
- **B** May be due to an abnormal fetus
- **C** Increases the risk of prolapse of the cord
- **D** Increases the risk of postpartum haemorrhage (PPH)
- **E** Causes an increased perinatal mortality due to asphyxia

A36 **Which of the following are true of the social security benefits for pregnant women in the United Kingdom?:**
- **A** A pregnant woman, who is entitled to Statutory Maternal Pay (SMP) should inform her employers 7 days before she intends to stop work
- **B** The form MAT B1(A) can be issued by the GP or midwife from 20 weeks
- **C** If a woman is not eligible for SMP, she may be entitled to the maternity allowance
- **D** If a woman claims maternity allowance after confinement, she should use form MAT B1(B)
- **E** Dental treatment is free for mothers up to 1 year after the baby is born

A37 **Acute pelvic inflammatory disease (PID):**
- **A** Is most commonly due to gonococcus in the UK
- **B** Can only be diagnosed accurately by laparoscopy
- **C** Gives an 8% risk of infertility after one attack
- **D** May follow spontaneous miscarriage
- **E** Requires tetracycline as part of treatment

A38 **Gestational diabetes mellitus:**
- **A** Will require insulin therapy if ketonuria develops on diet treatment
- **B** Is accurately screened for by urine testing for glucose
- **C** Can be screened for by serum fructosamine
- **D** Is diagnosed by a 100 g oral glucose tolerance test in the UK
- **E** Is more common in siblings of diabetics

A39 **Breastfeeding:**
- **A** Should be carried out every 4 hours
- **B** Should be stopped if mastitis occurs
- **C** Requires extra fluid intake for the mother
- **D** Should not start until 4 hours after delivery
- **E** Usually fails due to poor advice and lack of encouragement

A40 **Bleeding at 4 weeks post delivery:**
  A May be physiological
  B Is exacerbated by the progestogen-only pill
  C Is best treated by D&C
  D May be due to choriocarcinoma
  E May be due to carcinoma of the cervix

A41 **Neural tube defects (NTD) in pregnancy in the UK:**
  A The incidence is not geographically dependent
  B The risk of recurrence in subsequent pregnancies is 1 in 10
  C Are predominantly decreasing due to increased genetic counselling
  D Mainly occur in low-risk women
  E 95% of all women are now taking folic acid supplements in pregnancy

A42 **Recurrent miscarriages:**
  A 15% of women will suffer recurrent miscarriages
  B A balanced parental translocation is the most common cause of chromosomal abnormality
  C Is untreatable for antiphospholipid antibodies at present
  D Prognosis is poor for women with five miscarriages
  E Due to human chorionic gonadotrophin (hCG) is readily treatable

A43 **Progesterone-only post-coital contraception:**
  A Is more effective than Yupze regimens
  B Needs to be taken within 24 hours of unprotected intercourse
  C Is licensed for use in the UK
  D Has more side-effects than Yupze regimens
  E Two doses of 750 µg of levonorgestrel 12 hours apart are given with the first dose within 72 hours of unprotected intercourse.

A44 **Pregnancies in England:**
  A One in five pregnancies result in a termination
  B Abortion rates are independent of deprivation
  C Rates are decreasing
  D In 1995 a woman had 2.16 pregnancies during her lifetime
  E 40% of pregnancies in women under 20 are terminated

A45 **Care of near term infants with respiratory failure:**
  A Extracorpeal membrane oxygenation reduces mortality
  B Nitric oxide causes vasoconstriction
  C Meconium inactivates surfactant
  D Liquid ventilation is ineffective
  E Low frequency ventilation is useful

A46 Active management of the third stage of labour:
A Reduces the incidence of post-partum haemorrhage
B Increases the incidence of retained placenta
C Reduces the length of the third stage to a mean of 5 minutes
D Is less effective with an epidural in situ
E Involves giving 0.5 mg ergometrine with the anterior shoulder

A47 Causes of primary amenorrhoea include:
A Cryptomenorrhoea
B Turner's syndrome
C Polycystic ovary syndrome
D Lawrence–Moon–Biedl syndrome
E Testicular feminisation

A48 Acute retention of urine in women may be due to:
A Primary genital herpes
B Multiple sclerosis
C Ectopic ureter
D An ovarian cyst the size of a 20-week pregnancy
E Posterior colpoperineorrhaphy

A49 The following increase the risk of carcinoma of endometrium:
A An early menopause
B Maturity onset diabetes
C High parity
D Atypical endometrial hyperplasia
E Obesity

A50 Impending eclampsia is heralded by:
A Occipital headache
B Photophobia
C Epigastric pain
D Rising urate levels
E Fetal tachycardia

A51 Infection with *Listeria monocytogenes:*
A Causes mid-trimester miscarriage
B May present as pyelonephritis
C Causes meningitis in the neonate
D Is confirmed by culture of a high vaginal swab
E Is treated by doxycycline

A52 Pre-term rupture of the membranes at 30 weeks gestation is associated with:
A Painful contractions
B Breech presentation
C An abnormal fetus
D Chorioamnionitis
E Urinary tract infection

A53 **A normal 6-week infant:**
A Plays with his/her hands
B Has a positive Moro reflex
C Will only follow objects less than 12 inches away
D Will have had his/her first immunisation
E Has head control

A54 **Malignant disease of the vulva is associated with:**
A Atypical hyperplastic dystrophy
B Genital herpes infection
C Genital warts
D Lichen sclerosus
E Carcinoma of the cervix

A55 **Progestogen-only pills:**
A Have no thromboembolic risk
B Increase the risk of ectopic pregnancy
C Inhibit ovulation
D Make the cervical mucus more viscous
E Cause irregular menstruation

A56 **Detrusor instability:**
A Is rarely seen in general practice
B Commonly presents as nocturia
C Can only be diagnosed with certainty on urodynamic testing
D Can be treated by augmentation cystoplasty
E Will not respond to acupuncture

A57 **Genital tract infection with Chlamydia trachomatis:**
A May be asymptomatic
B Is associated with pre-term delivery
C May result in congenital pneumonia of the newborn
D Predisposes to salpingitis after vaginal termination of pregnancy
E Is easily diagnosed in general practice

A58 **A woman is discharged home on the 3rd day after a vaginal hysterectomy. She phones you 2 days later complaining of abdominal pain and vomiting. The possibilities include:**
A Pyelonephritis
B Vault infection
C Appendicitis
D Pulmonary embolism
E Constipation

A59 **A pregnant woman is requesting a home delivery and refuses to attend the hospital antenatal clinic. Her first delivery was by Caesarean section for fetal distress and the practice midwife requests your advice.**

A You are obliged to provide obstetric cover to the midwife if this goes ahead

B Your midwife can refuse to care for the woman if she labours at home

C The most likely outcome is a normal delivery

D The woman is at increased risk of placenta praevia

E A consultant obstetrician should be requested to do a domiciliary visit

A60 **The following statements concerning treatment of carcinoma of the ovary are true:**

A The prognosis depends on the amount of tumour remaining at the end of the first operation

B Stage Ia tumours require a 6-month course of methotrexate

C A second look laparotomy is required at 6 months

D Radiotherapy is effective

E Unilateral salpingo-oophorectomy is adequate for early stage dysgerminomas in young women

PAPER A
ANSWERS

A1 **A** **False** Blood pressure falls in the second trimester, then rises in the third trimester.

   B **True** A standard cuff (12 × 23 cm) will not encompass the arm of 5% of hypertensive pregnant patients. A large cuff must be used to avoid overdiagnosing hypertension in obese women.

   C **True** This position may cause supine hypotension, as the gravid uterus can impair venous return via the inferior vena cava. A semirecumbent position with lateral tilt and with the cuff at the same level as the heart will produce more accurate results.

   D **True** This is true predominantly for the second half of pregnancy. Only 2% of women will have a reading this high in the first half of pregnancy.

   E **False** In some pregnant women, the Korotkoff V phase can be heard at zero cuff pressure. For this reason, Korotkoff IV phase should be taken as the diastolic reading in pregnant women.

A2 **A** **False** Underweight primigravida are particularly affected. Other risk factors for pre-eclampsia include: a family history of pre-eclampsia, age under 20 or over 35, chronic hypertension and renal disease.

   B **True** The presence of these symptoms suggest that the woman is seriously ill with impending eclampsia.

   C **False** Smokers have a lower incidence of pre-eclampsia than non-smokers. However, smoking is associated with other adverse obstetric outcomes, e.g. low-birthweight babies.

   D **False** It causes asymmetrical growth retardation.

   E **False** There is no consensus as to which antihypertensive should be used. Methyl dopa and labetalol are most widely used. Nifedipine is not licensed for use in pregnancy although there are data to support its safety record.

A3 **A** **True** This abnormality in its most severe form leads to a single ventricle within the cranium, and is associated with midline facial abnormalities. There is always absence of the falx cerebri, which distinguishes it from *hydranencephaly*, in which the cranium is fluid-filled and brain tissue is absent.

B **True** *Gastroschisis* is a defect in the anterior abdominal wall. There is normal insertion of the umbilical cord, the hernia occurring usually to the right of the midline. The contents of the hernia have no covering membrane, as opposed to an *omphalocoele* which occurs through the umbilicus in the midline. The presence of an omphalocoele is associated with other midline abnormalities, and 50% have cardiac and chromosomal abnormalities. In both conditions, serum alpha fetoprotein is raised.

C **False** No anatomical markers exist for cystic fibrosis. It can now be diagnosed in some families by chorionic villus biopsy.

D **True** Posterior urethral valves occur almost exclusively in male infants, and cause varying degrees of dilatation of the urinary tract. Approximately 25% of affected fetuses will have a chromosome abnormality, and termination may be considered.

E **True** The early diagnosis of cardiac lesions ensures delivery in a specialist centre where treatable conditions can be dealt with urgently. Hypoplastic left heart is a fatal abnormality.

A4 **A** **False** Aminophylline has been used in pregnancy with no adverse effects on the fetus. It is important not to undertreat asthma or any other medical condition in pregnancy.

B **True** There is some risk of fetal growth retardation with regular steroid therapy in excess of 12 mg/day. It is unclear whether the cause of this growth retardation is arterial hypoxaemia or steroid therapy in pregnant women with severe asthma.

C **False** Status asthmaticus is uncommon during labour, and is thought to be protected against by high levels of endogenous catecholamines and corticosteroids.

D **True** The inheritance is polygenic.

E **False** Beta-sympathomimetic drugs, such as salbutamol, are safe for the fetus. They may cause maternal pulmonary oedema if given intravenously, but are safe if inhaled. They are used in the treatment of premature labour in non-asthmatics, but they do not seem to delay the onset of labour nor prolong labour in women with asthma.

A5 **A** **True** The last confidential enquiry (1994–1996) into maternal deaths in England and Wales lists pulmonary embolism and hypertension as the most frequent causes of maternal death. The incidence of pulmonary embolism is 5 times greater in pregnant than in non-pregnant women, the most dangerous period being the first 7 days of the puerperium. The Executive summary can be found on http: http://www.doh.gov.uk/cmo/mdeaths.htm.

B **False** Warfarin (a coumarin derivative) is teratogenic. The effects on the fetus include saddle nose, frontal bossing, midface hypoplasia, short stature, cardiac defects, mental retardation and blindness. Warfarin should be avoided in the first trimester and around the time of delivery. Patients with thrombosis and thromboembolism in pregnancy should be treated with intravenous heparin for 5–7 days, followed by intermittent subcutaneous heparin or warfarin depending on gestation.

C **False** 25–50% of patients with suspected venous thrombosis do not have thrombosis, therefore it is important to weigh the risks of unnecessary anticoagulation against the small potential risk of radiation. If venography is thought to be necessary, a lead apron shielding the pelvis gives protection to the fetus.

D **False** Local bruising, thrombocytopenia, over-anticoagulation, hypersensitivity reactions and bone demineralisation (osteoporosis) may all occur with subcutaneous heparin.

E **True** The risk of fatal pulmonary embolism is 10 times greater after Caesarean section than after vaginal delivery. Other factors found to be important by the confidential enquiries include: age, parity, excessive obesity, hospitalisation and restricted activity (especially if for an obstetric complication). Suppression of lactation by oestrogen, a history of previous DVT or PE, the presence of lupus anticoagulant and hereditary thrombotic disease are also risk factors. All women undergoing Caesarean section should be assessed for prophylaxic heparin against thromboembolism.

A6 **A** **True** The outcome relates to developing superimposed pre-eclampsia, but it is probably advisable to treat this level of hypertension for maternal reasons.

B **True** Weight gain is a poor predictor of outcome, and low weight is compatible with a normal-sized infant. The average weight gain in pregnancy is 10–12 kg, but many feel routine weighing in pregnancy could be abandoned.

C **True** This is usually physiological due to fluid retention and, to a lesser degree, obstruction from the gravid uterus.

D **False** Chronic renal failure has a poor outcome and most women will never become pregnant.

E **False** Few survive to childbearing age anyway, although modern therapy with iron-chelating agents does prolong survival.

A7 **A** **True** The mean minimum value accepted by the World Health Organization is 11.0 g/dl (at sea-level). For non-pregnant women, it is 12.0 g/dl. In the UK, haemoglobin levels below 10 g/dl in the second and third trimesters are likely to be abnormal and should be investigated.

B **False** In iron deficiency anaemia, there is a low serum iron and raised total iron binding capacity (TIBC), with a hypochromic microcytic film and a low serum ferritin. Chronic disorders, such as SLE and rheumatoid arthritis, produce an anaemia with a low serum iron and TIBC.

C **True** The increase in maternal red cell mass requires a net gain of 500–600 mg during pregnancy. 250–300 mg is also required for transfer to the fetus. The daily requirement is 3–4 times that of a non-pregnant woman.

D **True** The increased demand for iron is met by increasing the absorption of iron from the gut and by mobilisation of maternal stores.

E **True** The normal plasma volume of a non-pregnant woman is 2600 ml and increases in singleton pregnancies by 1250 ml. Most of the increase in volume occurs before 32 weeks of gestation. This increase is related to birthweight, and is greater in multiple pregnancy and in second and subsequent pregnancies.

A8 **A** **False** While a low Apgar score of 3 at 5 minutes post delivery is associated with an increased incidence of cerebral palsy, only 16% of those that survive have cerebral palsy. If the score is still 3 at 20 minutes, 57% will have cerebral palsy. However, it should be remembered that 75% of children with cerebral palsy have 5-minute Apgar scores of 7 or greater, and the strongest correlation with subsequent cerebral palsy is low birthweight (22 times more likely in infants below 1500 g compared to those over 2500 g).

B **False** Electronic fetal monitoring measures fetal asphyxia, but is a poor predictor of subsequent cerebral palsy. This may be because cerebral palsy may not be a consequence of perinatal asphyxia.

C **True** Other signs include: a rise or fall in temperature, drowsiness, vomiting, failure to gain weight, an anxious look and a greyish pallor of the skin. The commonest causative organisms are *Escherichia coli, Staphylococcus, Pseudomonas aeruginosa, Proteus* and *Haemolytic streptococcus.*

D **True** One in 500 infants will die suddenly and unexpectedly. The risk factors include: low birthweight, twin pregnancy, bottle-feeding, young mothers, illegitimacy, poor housing conditions, excessive cot covers and a prone sleeping position.

E **True** It is notifiable in the UK except in Northern Ireland.

A9 **A** **False** Autosomal dominant. Other examples of autosomal dominant disorders include: facioscapulohumeral dystrophy, Gilbert's syndrome, Marfan's syndrome, neurofibromatosis, osteogenesis imperfecta tarda, polycystic disease of the kidney (adult form), tuberous sclerosis and Von Willebrand's disease.

B **True** Enzyme defects tend to be autosomal recessive. Other examples include: albinism, congenital adrenal hyperplasia, cystic fibrosis, galactosaemia, Gaucher's disease, glycogen storage diseases, Tay-Sachs disease and Wilson's disease.

C **False** Tuberous sclerosis is inherited as an autosomal dominant. Clinical features include: adenoma sebaceum, subungual fibromas, shagreen patches and cafe-au-lait spots. Hamartomas, intracranial gliomas, cardiac rhabdomyomas and interstitial lung disease are also seen.

D **False** Huntingdon's chorea is inherited as an autosomal dominant, and usually presents after the age of 30. It causes choreiform movements associated with progressive dementia.

E **True** Retinitis pigmentosa causes progressive blindness from an early age, and most types are autosomal recessive. Autosomal dominant and X-linked recessive types do occur.

A10 **A** **True** Shoulder dystocia is a very serious and often totally unexpected complication of the second stage of labour. All personnel involved in intrapartum care must be able to recognise shoulder dystocia and take appropriate action. Big women have big babies, although the size of the fetus may be masked by the size of the mother.

B **True** Mid-cavity forceps is a risk factor, because it may represent some degree of disproportion as the fetal head has failed to pass the pelvic outlet.

C **True** Any condition leading to macrosomia increases the risk of shoulder dystocia (see **A**). In diabetics, the fetal head may be of normal size but the body is disproportionately large and the shoulders fail to enter the pelvis as the head is delivering.

D **True** The mean birthweight at 42 weeks is greater than at 40 weeks. Almost all the growth will have occurred by 40 weeks, and so it should not be deduced that elective delivery at 40 weeks would solve the problem.

E **False** Dysfunctional labour is due to poor uterine action. Secondary arrest of labour, particularly if response to oxytocin is poor, may indicate relative disproportion.

A11 **A** **True**   Although it need not mean the baby is distressed.

     B **True**   Any induction increases the risk of Caesarean section.

     C **True**   Although with fetal blood sampling this can be reduced.

     D **True**   This suggests disproportion or OP position.

     E **False** Cord prolapse is no more common than after spontaneous rupture.

A12 **A** **True**   PPH is defined as blood loss of more than 500 ml from the genital tract in the first 24 hours after delivery. An oxytocic given with delivery of the anterior shoulder, followed by controlled cord traction to deliver the placenta, will reduce the incidence of PPH.

     B **False** Uterine atony is the commonest cause of PPH (90%). Trauma accounts for 7%, and coagulation defects for the remaining 3%.

     C **False** Grand multiparity (4 or more births) predisposes to PPH. One reason may be an increasing amount of fibrous tissue within the uterine wall hindering effective contraction of the uterus.

     D **True**   These women should be booked for consultant delivery. Other factors predisposing to PPH include: uterine over-distension (e.g. polyhydramnios, multiple pregnancy), multiparity, antepartum haemorrhage and poor uterine action.

     E **True**   Delay in performing hysterectomy for PPH is a recurrent theme in the confidential enquiries into maternal death.

A13 **A** **False** There are about 2000 deaths due to cervical cancer annually in England and Wales (3% of cancer deaths in women). The average GP will see one new case every 5 years. Ovarian cancer kills twice as many women as cervical cancer, about 4000 deaths annually in England and Wales.

     B **True**   Cervical cancer is 5 times more common in social class V than it is in the professional classes. It is more common in urban than in rural areas.

C **True** The number of sexual contacts of a woman's partner has been found to be significant risk factor in the development of cervical cancer. Other risk factors include age of woman at first intercourse, a large number of sexual partners and lower socioeconomic group. The relationship with the human papilloma viruses is unclear, and there is no relationship with herpes virus type II. The relationship of cervical cancer to parity is unclear.

D **True** The death rate from cancer of the cervix continues to fall and the Health of the Nation target to reduce the incidence of invasive cervical cancer by at least 20% by the year 2000 has been met. This is largely due to a national screening programme that identifies women from the FHSA population register when they reach their 20th birthday and, at the end of 1993, 82.9% of eligible women had a cervical smear in the preceding 5 years.

E **True** It has been estimated that there may be a 10% false-negative rate. Necrotic tumours may result in negative cytology.

A14 **A** **False** Many sources suggest that use of the IUCD increases the risk of ectopic pregnancy. Any form of contraception reduces the incidence of pregnancy, and therefore of ectopic pregnancy. Permanent users of the IUCD have the same risk of ectopic pregnancy as those who have never used them, except with the no longer used Progestasert (a progesterone-releasing IUCD) which did increase the incidence of ectopics. However, if pregnancy does occur in a woman using an IUCD, the relative risk of an ectopic pregnancy is considerably increased. Pill users are at least risk (one-third the incidence with IUCDs). The aetiological factors identified for ectopic pregnancy are: pelvic inflammatory disease, increasing age, race (commoner in non-whites), previous tubal surgery or in vitro fertilisation (IVF), and a previous ectopic pregnancy.

B **False** The figure given in textbooks for the likelihood of an intra-uterine gestation and an ectopic pregnancy occurring simultaneously is 1 in 30 000. However, with an increasing prevalence of pelvic inflammatory disease and induced ovulation, recent American studies suggest the incidence is significantly higher, 1 in 7000. A 'pseudo-gestational sac' may be seen within the uterus in an ectopic pregnancy due to ectopic hormonal stimulation of the endometrium. This is seen in 10–20% of ectopic pregnancies on ultrasound scanning.

C **True** Only one-third of women with previous ectopics who wish to conceive will produce a live infant, and 10% will have another ectopic pregnancy.

D **True** Sensitive assays are now available which can always exclude early pregnancy. Older types of pregnancy testing involving agglutination techniques were less sensitive and so could be negative in the presence of an ectopic pregnancy.

E **True** These women tend to present late. Sterilisation should not be performed if the woman has had unprotected intercourse in the preceding 2 weeks.

A15 **A** **True** The vascular effects of the contraceptive pill are closely linked with cigarette smoking.

B **True** Although of minimal importance for healthy women. If they are used for diabetics, then careful review of their insulin requirements will be required.

C **False** Recent evidence is against this, and it appears equally as common in users of barrier contraception.

D **True** The oral contraceptive pill can be used for postcoital contraception within 72 hours of intercourse. Two 50 µg pills 12 hours apart will cause a withdrawal bleed within 21 days in 98% of women. It is important to confirm that this has occurred.

E **False** The combined oral contraceptive pill is highly protective against ovarian cancer, and this protection increases with use. The mechanism probably lies in the suppression of ovarian function.

A16

A **False** The equivalent amounts of oestrogen and progestogen in HRT are significantly less than those necessary in the combined pill in order to suppress ovulation. Consequently, the incidence of side-effects is less with HRT. Hormone replacement therapy does not lower the very high follicle-stimulating hormone (FSH) and luteinising hormone (LH) levels found in postmenopausal women to any degree.

B **True** The expected fracture rate of 40 fractures/1000 patient years is significantly reduced to only 3 fractures/1000 patient years, even in osteoporotic postmenopausal women.

C **True** Progestogens are given to women who have not had a hysterectomy. It protects against the risk of endometrial carcinoma, which is increased with unopposed oestrogens. However, progestogens may possibly reverse the beneficial effects of oestrogens on plasma lipids and lipoproteins.

D **True** A potential carcinogenic effect of HRT on the breast (which is known to be an oestrogen target organ) has not yet been proved. However, pre-existing breast cancer is an absolute contraindication to hormone replacement therapy. Other absolute contraindications include hormone-dependent cancers of the endometrium and ovary. Relative contraindications are: pre-existing hypertension, a history of thromboembolic disease, myocardial infarction, benign breast disease, diabetes, fibroids, gallbladder disease and familial hyperlipidaemia. It would seem sensible for GPs to ask specialists about women with these relative contraindications who have severe menopausal symptoms.

E **True** Oestrogens have a beneficial effect on the incidence of ischaemic heart disease in postmenopausal women, as compared to the adverse effect of oestrogens given in the combined oral contraceptive pill. This beneficial effect also applies to women who smoke. Progestogens are associated with an increased incidence of ischaemic heart disease. Some combinations have an overall worsening effect on lipids and the lipoprotein profile.

A17 **A** **False** The advantages of inserting the IUCD during menstruation or immediately after a period are that pregnancy is excluded, insertion is easy and any associated bleeding is accepted as normal loss. However, some women prefer not to be examined at this time.

B **False** It is important not to remove an IUCD until 1 year after the menopause. At present, it is recommended that Multiload Cu 250 and Mulitiload Cu 250 short are replaced after 3 years, Gynefix, Mirena and Multiload Cu 375 inert devices are changed every 5 years and Gyne T 380 every 10 years.

C **True** Provided intercourse has occurred no longer than 5 days previously, an IUCD will prevent implantation. Women should be reviewed after 1 month to check menstruation has occurred and to consider removal of the device.

D **True** Spontaneous abortion will occur in about 55% of cases (a 3 times greater incidence than in women without an IUCD). Removal of the IUCD may itself cause abortion, but if this does not happen it will reduce the risk of subsequent abortion. There is no evidence that copper-containing devices cause an increased incidence of fetal abnormality. The device is always extra-amniotic.

E **True** Insertion of an IUCD is not a sterile procedure, and the endometrium is colonised following insertion. The risk is higher in nulliparous women. Organisms implicated include chlamydia, gonococcus, anaerobes and, rarely, infection with *Actinomyces israeli*.

A18 **A** **True** Mean menstrual loss is 35 ml, with 95% of women losing less than 60 ml each menses. Menorrhagia is defined as a mean menstrual loss greater than 80 ml, or prolonged (greater than 7 days) menstrual loss. The passage of large clots and flooding indicates a large menstrual loss; however, the woman's own assessment of duration and number of sanitary pads or tampons used correlates poorly with actual blood loss. In about 50% of women with menorrhagia, no cause is found and it is referred to as dysfunctional uterine bleeding. Organic causes include congenital double uterus, IUCD, chronic pelvic inflammatory disease, uterine fibroids, uterine neoplasms and oestrogen-producing ovarian neoplasms. It is also seen with obesity, endometriosis and bleeding disorders.

B   True   Non-steroidal anti-inflammatory drugs are prostaglandin synthetase inhibitors. They can reduce menstrual loss by up to 30%. Unfortunately, the benefit decreases over several cycles. Other treatments include: antifibrinolytic agents, danazol, the combined oral contraceptive pill, hysteroscopic transcervical resection of the endometrium and hysterectomy.

C   False   Although the incidence of haemorrhage is increased in teenage girls and peri-menopausal women, over 50% are in the 20–40 year age group.

D   False   D&C is unlikely to be useful in the treatment of most cases of menorrhagia. It helps only in chronic anovulation (as it removes much of the hyperplastic endometrium) and for endometrial polyps and pedunculated leiomyomas of the uterus (fibroids). It is also useful diagnostically in women over 40 years of age to exclude endometrial carcinoma.

E   True   Medical treatment may be used in the interim. The reason for referral is to exclude a pathological cause. The GP should consider performing a full blood count (to exclude anaemia and thrombocytopenia) and a thyroid function test (to exclude hypothyroidism). Sudden changes in menstrual loss should be urgently investigated at this age.

A19   A   True   Although figures vary, female causes do seem to predominate. Male factors are being increasingly identified but are more difficult to treat. In many cases, there is a combined cause.

B   True   This is a useful test but the result comes several weeks after the event. Luteinising hormone assays are available and will predict ovulation within 12 hours. They are expensive and not routinely available, but commercial kits are available over the counter (e.g. Predictor).

C   True   The normal time to conceive increases with age, although it is reasonable to start investigations earlier in older couples.

D   True   A history of sub-fertility increases the risk of ectopic pregnancy. This is probably because it identifies a group of women with tubal problems.

E   True   Salazopyrin therapy for ulcerative colitis leads to oligospermia. It is reversible on stopping therapy.

A20 A True   Endometriosis is associated with infertility (30–45% of infertile women). Whether this is causal or casual is still debated. There is also an association with women who delay their first pregnancy. It is repeatedly stated in the literature that there is an increase in the higher socioeconomic groups, but this is unlikely to be a true association. There is also no evidence that women of Afro-Caribbean descent have a lower incidence of endometriosis. Inheritance is polygenic; 7% of first-degree relatives are affected compared to only 1% of unrelated controls.

B True   This is thought to be due to the greater mean menstrual blood loss with an IUCD, increasing from a normal amount of 35 ml up to 60 ml with small copper devices and 80 ml with a Lippes loop. This results in a greater volume of retrograde menstruation, one of the postulated aetiologies of endometriosis.

C True   Approximately 10% of women with endometriosis have involvement of the urinary tract. Other sites affected include the ovaries, pelvis, bowel, lower genital tract, the umbilicus and abdominal scars. The classic symptoms of endometriosis are cyclical pelvic pain and infertility.

D True   The pill needs to be taken continuously to produce amenorrhoea and 'pseudopregnancy'. The dose may have to be increased to up to 4 tablets per day, but this will produce increased side-effects. Other medical treatments include danazol, luteinising hormone releasing hormone (LHRH) agonists and Gestrinone, a new 19-nortestosterone derivative.

E True   HRT should be given to prevent immediate menopausal symptoms due to oestrogen deficiency, to prevent long-term osteoporosis and, possibly, to reduce the increased risk of ischaemic heart disease.

A21 A True   The risk of miscarriage once a live fetus has been seen on ultrasound is approximately 1 in 200.

B True   Abnormal karyotypes are found in approximately 50% of cases, the most common of which is autosomal trisomy (which accounts for 50%).

C **False** There is no evidence that progestogens reduce the risk of miscarriage despite their wide use in general practice. The proposed rationale for using them is that the corpus luteum is the principle source of progesterone during early pregnancy and luteal defects may lead to recurrent miscarriage. However, the lesson of diethylstilboestrol administration for recurrent miscarriage should not be forgotten. This treatment was found to be ineffective and caused vaginal adenocarcinoma in the offspring. There is some evidence that hCG may reduce the risk of recurrent miscarriage but it should not be used until further larger follow-up studies have been performed.

D **True** In the community, anti-D is difficult to obtain and, as a result, is often not given. If the rhesus factor of a patient is not known, then anti-D should be given as a matter of course (50 µg within the first 48 hours). Rhesus disease is preventable, and must not be ignored or forgotten.

E **True** Following incomplete abortion, ascending infection may occur. The early signs include raised temperature, abdominal pain, continued bleeding and an offensive vaginal discharge. If infection is suspected, the woman should be admitted to hospital, intravenous antibiotics administered and evacuation performed. Criminal abortion may still need to be considered.

A22 **A** **True**

B **True** The incidence of osteoporotic fractures may even increase before the menopause. It increases further with increasing age.

C **False** They rise to approach male levels, and this helps to explain the increased incidence of cardiovascular disease after the menopause.

D **False** It is well absorbed by the vagina and hence will have a systemic effect.

E **True** There is a very small increased risk of a DVT in the first year of use. This then disappears so that if a woman has not had one by 1 year her risk is back to baseline.

A23 **A** **True** There is usually abdominal distension from the tumour mass or from accompanying ascites. Ovarian tumours are characteristically symptomless in the early stages. Other recognised symptoms include: dysmenorrhoea, dyspareunia, increase in abdominal girth, increasing weight, acute abdominal pain, lower limb swelling, cachexia and dyspnoea.

 B **False** The mortality in social class I is twice that in social class V. There is also an association with nulliparity, breast cancer, exposure to talc and asbestos and previous pelvic irradiation. Previous mumps and the combined oral contraceptive pill are believed to have a protective effect. The overall incidence for women aged 45 is 1 in 10 000. There are genetic associations with the BRCA1 and BRCA2 genes. The relative risks of first-degree relatives also being affected are 3.8 for sisters, 6.0 for daughters and 11.7 for more than one affected relative (*Br J Obs Gynaecol* 1998; 105: 493–9).

 C **False** The majority of patients present as either stage III (growth involving one or both ovaries with intra-peritoneal metastases) or stage IV (growth involving one or both ovaries with distant metastases).

 D **True** Ovarian cancer accounts for 50% of all deaths from cancer of the female genital tract, but only 25% of gynaecological cancer. In spite of better cytotoxic treatment, the overall 5-year survival rate has changed little in recent years and remains at around 25–30%.

 E **False** The longer the pill is used, the less the likelihood of ovarian cancer. High parity, pregnancy (whether ending in abortion or at term), and breastfeeding all appear to be protective. An early menarche and a late menopause are associated with an increased risk. It appears that ovarian cancer is commoner in women who ovulate for longer.

A24 **A** **True** There is a direct positive correlation between the incidence of secondary amenorrhoea in runners and the number of miles run per week. As training becomes more strenuous, levels of LH and FSH fall significantly.

B **False** The majority of women resume ovulatory cycles within 4–6 weeks; however, it is not unusual for a woman to have 1 or 2 months of amenorrhoea before her first menstrual period. Investigation should be considered for more protracted amenorrhoea.

C **True** Amenorrhoea traumatica (Asherman's syndrome) may follow D&C, particularly if it has been performed in the puerperium. It is treated by breaking the adhesions via a hysteroscope and inserting an IUCD to keep the uterine walls apart.

D **True** Amenorrhoeic women have low levels of oestrogens and this will lead to osteoporosis even before the menopause. Treatment with the contraceptive pill should be considered.

E **False** FSH and LH will be raised as there will be no negative feedback on the hypothalamic-pituitary axis. The gonadotrophins are also increased in resistant ovary syndrome. Other investigations should include TSH, prolactin and visual field testing.

A25 **A** **True** Pre-term delivery is defined as delivery before 37 weeks of gestation. Other risk factors include: parity of one or more than four, social class, previous pre-term delivery, antepartum haemorrhage, multiple pregnancy and, possibly, genital tract infection. Asymptomatic bacteriuria in the absence of renal involvement does not appear to increase the risk of a pre-term delivery. Prevention has thus been largely unsuccessful and the incidence has not changed in recent years.

B **False** There is no increased risk providing there is atraumatic cervical dilatation. However, second trimester abortions and stillbirths are risk factors.

C **False** Almost any severe maternal illness may be associated with pre-term delivery. Diabetes mellitus is associated with polyhydramnios, congenital abnormalities, hypertension and renal disease.

D **False** Although effective treatment for cervical incompetence, cerclage has not been shown to be an effective method of preventing pre-term labour in women at risk.

E **True** Most cases of painful contractions settle spontaneously, and tocolytic therapy is unnecessary. The problem is trying to identify the minority who will go on to deliver. If rupture of the membranes has occurred, then pre-term delivery will occur in the vast majority.

A26 **A** **False** Not in themselves, although if the parents allow the use of steroids or transfer to a neonatal intensive care unit then they will be of help.

B **True** They affect the fetal cardiovascular system and can lead to neonatal hyperglycaemia.

C **True** Maternal deaths have occurred, particularly if the drugs are given in large volumes of intravenous fluids.

D **False** They are the drugs of choice. Beta blockers are potentially dangerous in asthmatics.

E **True** Blood sugar must be monitored, and the drugs are relatively contraindicated in diabetics. If they are used, alteration of insulin dosage will be required.

A27 **A** **False** It is only mid-trimester termination that may lead to subsequent miscarriage. Serial examinations are not helpful and a decision regarding a cervical suture should be taken at booking.

B **True** Essential for mother, baby and attendants.

C **True** Thalassaemia is common, and prenatal diagnosis is offered if both partners have thalassaemia trait. Women with this condition will have a low haemoglobin and should not be given parenteral iron.

D **False** The initial promise from uncontrolled studies has not been confirmed by controlled studies. Problems include: extra workload from performing the CTGs, the anxiety induced in the mothers and difficulty in interpretation of antenatal CTGs.

E **True** Although not necessary for healthy mothers with singleton pregnancies, iron and folate supplements are recommended for twin pregnancies.

A28 A True The main problems of HIV infection in pregnancy are that pregnancy may aggravate the course of the disease, and that the disease is transmissible from the mother to the fetus.

B True Transplacental transmission occurs early in pregnancy. The reported fetal abnormalities include: growth failure, 'box' forehead, wide-set eyes, short nose and patulous lips.

C True The exact risk is not known, but HIV-positive mothers should be advised to bottle-feed.

D True *Cryptococcus neoformans* is the commonest cause of meningitis, bacterial causes being uncommon. If the treatment required is teratogenic, termination should be considered. Other overwhelming opportunistic infections found include: *Toxoplasma gondii*, *Cryptosporidium*, *Strongyloides*, *Pneumocystis carinii*, *Herpes simplex*, *Salmonella*, *Aspergillus* and *Mycobacterium avium* and *intracellulare*.

E True Other tumours associated with HIV infection are Kaposi's sarcoma and Hodgkin's and non-Hodgkin's lymphoma.

A29 A True Club foot is one of the commonest congenital malformations, occurring in 1 per 1000 live births. Male infants are twice as commonly affected as females (M:F = 2:1). Orthopaedic opinion should be sought, and application of plaster boots recommended, at an early stage. Despite these measures, surgery is necessary in 30% of affected infants before the age of 11.

B False 90% of affected infants are female (M:F = 1:9). Other risk factors include: a positive family history (in 20%), breech delivery (incidence 10 times higher) and first-born babies. The incidence is approximately 15 per 10 000 live births. The left hip is affected twice as often as the right. Splinting should commence at 36 hours after birth and be continued for at least 2 months. The orthopaedic surgeon will be involved from an early stage.

C   **True**   Over 80% of affected infants are male (M:F = 5:1). The incidence is 2 per 1000 live births. The risk increases if there is a family history. It should be considered in any infant under 3 months of age presenting with recurrent vomiting. It is suspected clinically by the presence of a palpable abdominal mass during or after a test feed, and the diagnosis may be confirmed by ultrasound or by a barium meal. Treatment is by surgery.

D   **False**   Isolated cleft palate is commoner in females, but cleft palate associated with cleft lip is commoner in males. In 30% of affected infants there is a positive family history. Other risk factors include certain drugs used in pregnancy, such as warfarin and steroids. Considerable parental support is needed, both with counselling and practical aspects of feeding. The lip is normally repaired from the 1st to the 12th week of life, with later repair of the palate at 9 months. Early involvement of a speech therapist is useful.

E   **True**   80% of affected infants are male (M:F = 4:1). The incidence is 1 in 5000 live births, but the condition may take several months to present. The infant is constipated as a result of an aganglionic segment of rectum or colon. Diagnosis can be made by barium enema and confirmed by absence of ganglion cells in a rectal biopsy. Surgical treatment involves resection of the aganglionic segment of large bowel.

A30   **A**   **False**   Jaundice appearing in the first 24 hours of life is never physiological. The commonest cause will be haemolytic disease. Other causes include congenital infection, maternal drug use, metabolic disorders and biliary atresia.

      B   **False**   This level of bilirubin is rarely reached in healthy, term babies. The liver of pre-term infants is less mature and the serum bilirubin will rise much quicker. Treatment will be required sooner.

      C   **False**   A positive Coomb's test will lead to haemolysis and then jaundice.

      D   **False**   Although extra fluids may be required to avoid dehydration there is no need to insist on full bottle-feeding.

      E   **True**   Jaundice affects virtually all pre-term babies to some degree. This is because of the relatively immature liver.

A31 **A** **False** Cyclical ovarian hormonal effects still persist with intact ovaries. However, the exact aetiological cause of pre-menstrual syndrome is not clear.

B **True** Support from the medical profession is very important if the woman is to be helped. Medical treatment is unlikely to work without a sympathetic doctor who acknowledges the woman's problems. Counselling and self-help groups are useful.

C **True** Aldosterone antagonists are helpful in women whose principle symptoms relate to fluid retention. They do not have any beneficial effect on mood. Spironolactone is usually given in a dose of 25 mg per day from day 18 to day 26 of the cycle. Other treatments include pyridoxine (for mood changes), natural progesterone (for emotional distress and physical symptoms), bromocriptine (for breast tenderness), danazol and diet. LHRH-agonists have been used in refractory cases, but they can only be used for short periods because of the anti-oestrogen effect.

D **False** It is defined as cyclical and as having a consistent and predictable relationship to the menses.

E **True** The oral contraceptive pill can aggravate symptoms in some women, whilst curing others. It is probably the continuous progestogen use that aggravates PMS and it should therefore be used with caution.

A32 **A** **True** Women initially have irregular uterine bleeding but most develop complete amenorrhoea. One-third are amenorrhoeic within 1 year. Depoprovera is not licensed for use in the USA, partly because an increased incidence of breast cancer has been found in beagles. This association has not been found in humans. In the USA, Depoprovera is used in the treatment of endometriosis and endometrial cancer.

B **False** It is recommended for use in women with sickle cell anaemia. The disease actually improves, with fewer sickle crises and a rise in serum haemoglobin. Oestrogens are contraindicated in sickle cell anaemia.

C True Medroxyprogesterone (150 mg i.m., 3-monthly) is probably even more effective than the combined oral contraceptive pill. Care must be taken to ensure that the woman is not pregnant before starting the treatment. Its main disadvantages are irregular menstruation initially, weight gain and some delay (up to 18 months) in the restoration of ovulation when the treatment is discontinued.

D True Minute amounts are excreted in breast milk, but no adverse effects have been found. In fact, there is evidence to suggest that the quality and quantity of milk produced is increased.

E True It is important to warm patients of this possible problem.

A33 A True Chorionic villus biopsy is becoming more widely available for prenatal diagnosis. Although its main advantage is that it can be used in the first trimester, it can still be used after 12 weeks. A technician is available to confirm that enough tissue has been obtained.

B True
RFLP Cystic fibrosis can be diagnosed on chorionic villi by restriction fragment length polymorphism. This requires genetic material from the two carriers (i.e. parents) and from the previously affected child.

C True DNA analysis of villi can diagnose male fetuses affected by haemophilia.

D True Chromosome analysis of the villi can usually be done within 24 hours, as the cells do not need to be cultured. Since this condition is commoner in women over 35, it may be diagnosed if CVS is done for this reason.

E True Fragile X is the most common cause of mental retardation in males after Down's syndrome. When fragile X mental retardation has been established within a family, prenatal testing should be carried out on at-risk fetuses.

A34 A False 4%, i.e. 1 in 25. The background incidence of spina bifida is 2 per 1000 births. Other causes of raised maternal serum AFP include: anencephaly, fetal anterior wall defects, congenital nephrosis, posterior urethral valves, Turner's syndrome, trisomy 13, oesophageal atresia, duodenal atresia, miscarriage and intra-uterine death.

B **True** Women with insulin-dependent diabetes tend to have low maternal serum AFP and a high risk of pregnancy affected by a neural tube defect. A cut-off lower than that in the general population is used in this group of women.

C **False** Fetuses with Down's syndrome produce less AFP than normal. This can be used to estimate the risk of Down's, which increases with advancing maternal age. It is 1 in 350 at 35 years, 1 in 100 at 40 years and 1 in 30 at 45 years.

D **True** This is performed to confirm gestational age and to look for the causes of a raised serum AFP. Often, a repeat AFP is performed before amniocentesis. The risks to the fetus must be considered before amniocentesis is carried out. In experienced hands, there is an estimated excess risk of 0.8% of fetal loss due to this procedure.

E **True** Intra-uterine death is associated with very high serum AFP levels. Vaginal bleeding early in pregnancy is also associated with high serum AFP, even if the pregnancy does not end in miscarriage.

A35 **A** **True** Approximately 2–3% of babies present by the breech at term. This incidence is not altered by external cephalic version unless it is performed after 38 weeks.

B **True** This is important if considering elective Caesarean section, and an ultrasound should be performed for fetal anomaly if not previsouly done.

C **True** The rate of cord prolapse with breech presentations is about 4%. This is mainly due to the increased incidence with flexed and footling breeches. The rate for extended breech presentation is similar to vertex presentations (0.3%).

D **False** There is no link with PPH per se. Obviously, the blood loss will be greater if Caesarean section is required.

E **True** Although there used to be a significant perinatal mortality from trauma in breech deliveries, this was mainly due to the practice of breech extraction. This has been abandoned (except for the second twin) and hence traumatic deaths are rare.

A36 **A** **False** The employer must be informed at least 21 days before the woman intends to leave work. The woman should supply the employer with the medical evidence of when the baby is due. This is in the form of a certificate (MAT B1), which is supplied by either the GP or the midwife. Full information is given in leaflet FB8, 'Babies and Benefits', obtainable from a social security office.

 B **False** The form MAT B1(A) is issued by the GP or midwife not earlier than 14 weeks before the expected week of delivery (i.e. after 26 weeks of pregnancy).

 C **True** This will depend on her National Insurance contributions. The woman should inform the DSS and supply them with the completed MAT B1 and MA1 forms. If she is employed, she should also submit a form SMP 1 from her employer stating why the employer will not pay SMP. Maternity allowance (as with SMP) is paid for 18 weeks starting from the 11th week before the baby is due.

 D **True** MAT B1(A) is used before confinement and form MAT B1(B) after confinement. If the woman cannot get either SMP from her employer or maternity allowance from social services she is still able to receive sickness benefit. The form MAT B1(A) is accepted as evidence of incapacity for work for the period starting 6 weeks before the birth of the baby, and ending 2 weeks after the actual date of the birth.

 E **True** NHS prescriptions are also free.

A37 **A** **False** *Chlamydia trachomatis* now appears to have taken over in the UK and in Scandinavia. Both organisms are often present together, and the rule that when one sexually transmitted disease is found others should be looked for applies. *Gonococcus* and *Chlamydia* are also the causes of the uncommon 'Fitz–Hugh–Curtis syndrome' of peri-hepatitis. In this syndrome, there is an exudative inflammation of the liver capsule secondary to pelvic infection. It can mimic acute cholecystitis.

 B **True** The main differential diagnosis of bilateral pelvic tenderness is endometriosis, which can only be excluded by laparoscopy. Laparoscopy also allows checking of tubal patency.

C **True** Other sequelae of PID include chronic pelvic pain, dyspareunia, menorrhagia, dysmenorrhoea and ectopic pregnancy (an increased risk of up to 10-fold).

D **True** The placental site is an ideal culture medium for infecting organisms. The usual organisms in this situation are *Escherichia coli*, *Clostridia*, *Streptococci* and *Staphylococci*.

E **True** No single drug covers all the organisms involved. The choice of antibiotic regimen depends on the likely cause. Culture for *Chlamydia* may take several days and is best presumed to be present unless proven otherwise. Tetracycline is the treatment of choice and should be continued for at least 14 days.

Chlamydiae = tetracycline

A38 **A** **False** Mild ketoacidosis is often found in diabetic pregnant women treated by diet alone and is not regarded as harmful. Gestational diabetes is usually treated with diet alone. Regular blood sugars should be monitored by the woman and the antenatal clinic. If diet fails to control blood sugars, insulin therapy should be added. Oral hypoglycaemic agents cross the placenta and induce fetal hyperinsulinaemia.

B **False** Glycosuria is very common in pregnancy due to less efficient renal tubular re-absorption. Blood sugar estimations are required to accurately screen for diabetes; they can be performed at random times and the results interpreted with reference to the last meal (e.g. 6.4 mmol/l less than 2 hours after a meal or 5.8 mmol/l at any other time).

C **False** Fructosamine and glycosylated haemoglobin (Hb A$_1$) are used to monitor control in insulin-dependent diabetics but are not suitable as a screening test. They indicate past levels of serum glucose rather than present levels.

D **False** Although 100 g tests are used in the USA, British, European and WHO criteria for the diagnosis of diabetes require a 75 g oral glucose tolerance test.

E **True** Other risk factors for gestational diabetes include fasting glycosuria, polyhydramnios and a previous history of gestational diabetes, macrosomia or unexplained stillbirth.

A39 **A** **False** Babies who are allowed to feed on demand put on more weight and continue breastfeeding longer. Interestingly, there is no increased incidence of cracked nipples with longer duration of feeds.

B **False** Breastfeeding should be continued, with particular attention given to correct positioning of the baby. Mastitis is best treated with flucloxacillin (500 mg orally qds for 5 days). The condition results from excess collections of milk in the breast alveoli, and can progress to infection and abcess formation. When this occurs, the woman develops systemic symptoms with shivering attacks, rigors, headaches and flu-like symptoms.

C **False** There is no evidence that increased fluid intake improves lactation. In fact, the increased urine output may cause distress to women with perineal and labial trauma.

D **False** There is no evidence that starting breastfeeding later (4 hours after the birth) is better or worse than starting early (immediately after delivery). It is more important that the women receive appropriate and practical help and support.

E **True** Although the evidence is not totally consistent, the duration of breastfeeding has been shown to be increased in women who have regular and frequent contacts with appropriate carers.

A40 **A** **True** It is likely to be physiological. The mean duration of lochia is 33 days, with 13% of women still having persistent lochia at 60 days. If bleeding continues to decrease progressively, it is likely to be normal.

B **True** The progestogen-only pill (POP) causes more breakthrough bleeding the earlier in the puerperium it is used, and for this reason may be discontinued by the woman. 50% fewer women discontinue treatment because of bleeding problems if the POP is commenced at 6 weeks post-partum compared with women who started it at 1 week post-partum. However, to reduce the risk of early fertile ovulation it is probably best started in the 3rd to 4th week of the puerperium.

C False If the bleeding is significant and increasing, a gynaecological opinion should be sought. Endometrial pathology is rare at 4 weeks, since retained products and infection will usually have presented by then. Curettage may occasionally be required, but must be performed by an experienced operator since perforation is more common than in the non-pregnant.

D True This is excessively rare 4 weeks post delivery.

E True The incidence is difficult to assess; however, the cervix must always be visualised.

A41 A False Neural tube defects in the west of Scotland are twice the national average, possibly due to low dietary folic acid.

B False The relative risk is 1 in 25.

C False There has been a 46% reduction of NTD between 1964 and 1988, compared with an 18% reduction in the number of births. Screening and improvements in dietary folic acid as well as folic acid supplements have had significantly larger contributions.

D True 95% of neural tube defects occur in low-risk women, but the risk is lower in women with no past obstetric history.

E False Figure in all studies are lower usually about 60%. There remains considerable scope for improvement particularly in unplanned pregnancies.

A42 A False 2% of women suffer recurrent miscarriages. There is no ethnic variation, although systemic lupus erythematous is 3 times more common in women of Afro-Caribbean descent.

B True This abnormality is found in 5% of patients. 50% of all spontaneously aborted fetuses have chromosome abnormalities. The percentage is increased with the earlier the miscarriage. Couples benefit from genetic counselling.

C **False** 15% of women with repeated loss have positive results for antiphospholipid antibodies (includes lupus anticoagulant and anticardiolipin antibodies). Low-dose aspirin (75 mg daily) results in birth rate of 42%. This rate is improved to 71% when aspirin is combined with low molecular weight heparin. Intravenous immunoglobulin is expensive and is no more effective. Intravenous leucocyte immunisation has not proved to be successful.

D **False** Even with treatment 50% of women who have had five miscarriages or more will have a live birth. Whilst this is a high eventual rate, women need comfort, support and as much explanation for the causes of miscarriage.

E **False** hCG deficiency may cause low progesterone concentration after implantation. hCG is thought to support the luteal phase and prolong the life of the corpus luteum. However, treatment with hCG does not appear to work except in women who have had a history of oligomennorrhoea. Other endocrine causes are corpus luteum deficiency and polycystic ovary syndrome. Neither hypothyroidism nor hyperthyroidism is associated with miscarriage.

A43 **A** **True** A WHO study of 2000 women showed a failure rate of 0.4% within 24 hours of unprotected sex compared with 2% with PC4. The failure rate increases to 2% between 49 and 72 hours post coital.

B **False** It needs to be taken within 72 hours but failure rate is less the earlier it is started.

C **False** At present it can only be given on a named patient basis with clear discussion about risks versus benefits with women giving informed consent.

D **False** Vomiting and other side-effects are reduced but can still occur.

E **True** At present this means 25 tablets and a further 25 tablets 12 hours later.

A44 **A** **True** In 1995 a mean lifetime abortion rate of 0.44 per woman. Most women are under 30 years of age, single and childless.

B **False** Contraceptive use is associated with social class and abortion rates rise with deprivation rate.

C **False** Rates are increasing with more women having repeat abortions.

D **True**

E **True** 20% of abortions occur in women under 20 years.

A45 **A** **True** Extracorpeal membrane oxygenation is considerably effective if started early. A double lumen catheter is placed into the right atrium and blood is drained, heated, oxygenated and reinjected into the same chamber.

B **False** Nitric oxide vasodilates and directly effects pulmonary vascular resistance. It improves matching of ventilation and perfusion without systemic effects.

C **True** Surfactant metabolism is important in respiratory disease in these infants as pneumonia, hypoplastic lungs and meconium all reduce the amount of surfactant.

D **False** Using fluorocarbon liquid in the lungs expands atelectic areas and redistributes blood flow. It supports gas exchange whilst lungs are recovering and may allow administration of drugs such as surfactant. It may be useful in infants with congenital diaphragmatic hernia. The evidence is at present limited.

E **False** High frequency ventilation may help in decreasing arterial carbon dioxide pressures but there are no reducible data yet to show improved outcome.

A46 **A** **True** The benefits of routine administration of oxytocics and controlled cord traction for the third stage of labour have been clearly shown.

B **True** Although the increase is small in comparison with the marked reduction in post-partum haemorrhage. The main problem is that an anaesthetic is required.

C **True** A passively managed third stage can last 20 minutes or longer.

D **False** An epidural has no influence on the third stage.

E **False** In most units, a combination of 5 units oxytocin and 0.5 mg ergometrine is given intramuscularly (1 ampoule of Syntometrine). Oxytocin alone should be used for women who are hypertensive or have cardiac disease.

A47 **A** **True** This is due to blockage to the outflow of menstrual blood and is usually caused by an imperforate hymen. It is easily treated by incising the membrane.

B **True** The diagnosis has sometimes been made before puberty and withdrawal bleeding will occur with hormone replacement. Many cases present with primary amenorrhoea as the only symptom.

C **False** Polycystic ovarian disease usually presents with irregular periods, anovulation and hirsutism.

D **True** This is due to a rare hypothalamic-pituitary disturbance and will have been diagnosed in childhood (mental retardation, retinitis pigmentosa and polydactyly).

E **True** Although genetically male, these patients are female in all other ways and should be treated as such. The testes are usually in the inguinal canal and should be removed to prevent malignant change.

A48 **A** **True** Primary infection with genital herpes is very painful and often made worse by secondary bacterial infection. The resulting acute retention is best relieved by supra-pubic catheterisation.

B **True** Retention of urine (other than after surgery or childbirth) is very rare, and neurological causes must be excluded. In practice, multiple sclerosis more commonly causes urinary frequency.

C **False** This causes incontinence because it usually opens below the bladder neck in women.

D **False** A cyst of this size would not impact on the pelvis and hence will not cause retention. It is likely to cause frequency and a feeling of incomplete emptying.

E **True** A common complication of vaginal surgery. Supra-pubic catheterisation is often preferred post-operatively because it avoids repeated catheterisation.

A49 **A** **False** A late menopause is a risk factor, possibly due to a longer exposure to endogenous oestrogens.

B **True**

C **False** Parous women have a lower risk of endometrial and ovarian cancer.

D **True** This carries an estimated 20% risk of endometrial cancer and hence hysterectomy is indicated. Simple cystic hyperplasia can be treated with cyclical progestogens, and has a less than 1% risk of developing into carcinoma.

E **True** Oestrogen is produced in adipose tissue and hence obese women may have relatively high levels. Needless to say, other factors must also be involved.

A50 **A** **False** Frontal headache is a characteristic feature of impending eclampsia, although other causes of headache may need to be considered (e.g. migraine).

B **True** Women with suspected pre-eclampsia should have fundoscopy to exclude the presence of papilloedema.

C **True** Epigastric pain is a serious symptom in pre-eclamptic women and is due to liver oedema and stretching of the capsule.

D **False** Although this may be a feature of worsening pre-eclampsia, it is not related to the risk of eclampsia. Women can be seriously ill with pre-eclampsia and never have a fit. Urate levels are used to assess the degree of renal impairment in pre-eclampsia, and levels have been shown to correlate with perinatal outcome.

E **False** There is no correlation with the fetal heart rate.

A51 **A** **True** It is an uncommon cause of miscarriage but is potentially preventable. Listeria contaminates soft cheeses, unpasteurised milk and, more recently, some 'cook-chill' foods.

B **True** A non-specific febrile illness and loin pain are early features.

C **True** It therefore has a high mortality unless recognised and treated early.

D **False** Blood cultures are required to make the diagnosis.

E **False** High-dose ampicillin is the treatment of choice.

A52 **A** **True** Pre-term labour and delivery occur within a week in most cases of pre-term rupture of the membranes.

B **True** Premature babies account for 25% of babies born breech. Delivery is often by Caesarean section if the baby is considered viable and believed to weigh less than 1.5 kg.

C **True** Abnormal babies often deliver prematurely.

D **True** Once this has occurred, delivery must be expedited for maternal and fetal reasons. Antibiotics should be started.

E **False** However, genital tract infection may have an aetiological role. Whether this is cause or effect is uncertain.

A53 **A** **False** They may begin to find their hands by this age, but do not generally start to play with them for another few weeks.

B **True** This would be present until about 3 months of age. Sudden movement of the neck initiates rapid abduction and extension of the arms and opening of the hands. The arms then come together.

C **True** Infants of this age can follow objects very close to their face that move from side to side. Their eyes do not show focusing and convergence until 8 weeks.

D **False** The new schedule starts diphtheria, tetanus and polio at 8 weeks, but there is evidence that immunisation can begin soon after birth.

E **False** Some minor degree of support is exhibited, but not proper head control. Head lag on pulling to a sitting from a lying position is normal.

A54 **A** **True** There are many types of vulval dystrophy and the classification has recently been modified. Any evidence of cellular atypia increases the risk of subsequent carcinoma, and careful follow-up is required.

B **False** This has no link with subsequent malignant change.

C **True** Although warts are common and carcinoma rare, there is a well-recognised association.

D **False** There is no association between lichen sclerosus and vulval carcinoma.

E **True** Whether the wart virus is the link remains uncertain, but women with carcinoma of the cervix have an increased risk of developing carcinoma of the vulva later.

A55 **A** **True** Progestogens are not linked to venous thrombosis. They are, however, linked with arterial disease (including hypertension). Newer progestogens, e.g. desogestrel, may have a lower risk.

    B **True** The risk is small and probably due to an effect on tubal motility.

    C **False** Although this may occur, the mechanism of its contraceptive action is its effect on the endometrium and cervical mucus.

    D **True** This makes it much more difficult for spermatozoa to penetrate the mucus.

    E **True** This remains the main disadvantage of this form of contraception.

A56 **A** **False** Detrusor instability affects up to 10% of women. Its incidence increases with age and accounts for an increasing proportion of elderly incontinent women.

    B **False** Frequency and urgency are the commonest symptoms. The prevalence of nocturia is related to age.

    C **True** Detrusor instability is a urodynamic diagnosis, particularly as sensory urgency presents in a similar way. However, not all women require this test before a trial of medical treatment.

    D **True** This is a useful treatment in selected women with severe symptoms.

    E **False** Hypnotherapy and acupuncture are useful adjuncts but not always available.

A57 **A** **True** This is the likely reason for the adverse effect of this infection on fertility. Sexually active women attending with discharge should be tested and the feasibility of screening is being investigated.

    B **True**

    C **True**

    D **True** Women undergoing termination should be screened or treated. This has been shown to reduce the risk of pelvic infection, ectopic pregnancy and infertility.

    E **False** Special culture fluid is required and needs to be refrigerated.

A58 **A** **True**

B **True** With earlier discharge from hospital, patients may develop complications after going home. Urinary tract and vaginal vault infections do still occur although the risk is reduced by prophylactic antibiotics used at the time of surgery.

C **True** Unrelated conditions can also occur after hysterectomy and of course after childbirth.

D **False** Pulmonary embolism will present with shortness of breath or haemoptysis.

E **True** Constipation is common after hysterectomy and may often be prevented by aperients as necessary.

A59 **A** **False**

B **False**

C **True**

D **True**

E **False**

A60 **A** **True** Whether this is a reflection on the surgeon or the tumour remains unclear. The first operation should remove as much tumour as possible and, in order to maximally debulk ovarian cancer, bowel resection may be required.

B **False** This has been shown to be unnecessary and runs the risk of causing a second tumour, i.e. leukaemia.

C **False** This does not in itself confer a survival advantage and there is at present no effective second-line treatment if a full course of chemotherapy has been given.

D **False** It may have a role as an adjuvant in stage Ic disease, but ovarian tumours (except dysgerminomas) are more susceptible to chemotherapy than to radiotherapy.

E **True** Several successful pregnancies have been reported after treatment for early stage dysgerminoma. Pelvic clearance is usually recommended once their family is complete.

PAPER B
QUESTIONS

B1 **Which of the following are features of the polycystic ovary syndrome?:**
- **A** Multiple pregnancies
- **B** Hair loss
- **C** Virilisation
- **D** Anorexia nervosa
- **E** Menorrhagia

B2 **Regarding termination of pregnancy in the UK:**
- **A** The majority are done under Section 1 of the 1967 Abortion Act
- **B** Vacuum aspiration is safer the later the gestation
- **C** ' A GP who has a conscientious objection may opt out of referring a woman for an abortion
- **D** It is illegal to refer and perform an abortion on a minor without parental consent
- **E** Women presenting for termination have often had a previous termination

B3 **The following conditions suggest that booking in a GP unit would be unwise:**
- **A** Previous hysterotomy
- **B** Previous PPH
- **C** Previous lift-out forceps delivery
- **D** A previous D&C
- **E** An 18-year old primigravida

B4 **Placental abruption:**
- **A** Is a less common cause of third trimester bleeding than placenta praevia
- **B** Is always due to rupture of spiral arteries beneath the placenta
- **C** Is predisposed to by cocaine abuse in pregnancy
- **D** The risk of recurrence is greater in smokers
- **E** May be recognised on ultrasound

B5 *Trichomonas vaginalis* **vaginal infection:**
- **A** Is usually sexually transmitted
- **B** Often occurs with gonorrhoea
- **C** Is treated with penicillin
- **D** Can be diagnosed by a characteristic ammonia smell when the discharge is mixed with 10% potassium chloride
- **E** Does not require treatment

B6 **Antepartum haemorrhage (APH):**
- **A** Is defined as bleeding from the genital tract after 20 weeks' gestation
- **B** Can be caused by cervical polyps
- **C** Can be managed at home if the bleeding is slight ✗ *Kleihauer*
- **D** Increases the risk of a PPH
- **E** Should have a vaginal digital examination performed immediately

B7 **Asymptomatic bacteriuria during pregnancy:**
- **A** Does not usually require any treatment
- **B** Requires investigation by intravenous urography (IVU) after delivery
- **C** Occurs in 5% of pregnant women ✓
- **D** Is usually caused by beta haemolytic streptococci
- **E** May lead to pyelonephritis

B8 **In the management of a prolapsed umbilical cord occurring at home which of the following statements are true?:**
- **A** No intervention should be attempted until the arrival of the flying squad
- **B** The condition is more common with twins
- **C** The cord should be placed gently back into the vagina
- **D** Catheterisation to empty the woman's bladder should be performed
- **E** The woman should be stood upright to aid immediate delivery

B9 **Prostaglandin PGE$_2$ intravaginal pessaries used in the induction of labour:**
- **A** Should be placed in the cervical canal
- **B** Do not promote cervical ripening in women with low Bishop scores
- **C** May induce fetal distress
- **D** Should be continued indefinitely until artificial rupture of the membranes (ARM) can be performed
- **E** May produce uterine hypertonia

B10 **Premature rupture of membranes:**
  A Is defined as the leakage of amniotic fluid prior to the onset of contractions at any stage of pregnancy up to 40 weeks
  B Amniotic fluid is detected by turning nitrazine yellow ⟶ blue
  C Digital vaginal examination must be performed
  D Prophylactic antibiotics decrease neonatal infections
  E Corticosteroids are contraindicated because of the risk of infection

B11 **Constipation in pregnancy:**
  A Is a result of delayed gastrointestinal motility
  B Liquid paraffin is contraindicated
  C Should not be treated with Senna
  D May cause acute abdominal pain
  E Is exacerbated by iron therapy

B12 **Concerning puberty in girls:**
  A The hypothalamus plays a major role in the onset of puberty
  B The appearance of pubic hair is the first sign
  C The average age of the menarche has fallen 12·5
  D Breast development usually starts by 11 years of age
  E Most cases of precocious puberty are pathological (boys)

B13 **Which of the following conditions are contraindications to the combined oral contraceptive pill?**
  A Varicose veins ✗
  B Otosclerosis ✓
  C Family history of diabetes mellitus ✓
  D Breastfeeding ✗ relative CI
  E Depression ✗   "   "

B14 **Laparoscopic sterilisation:**
  A In the UK, requires consent from both the husband and wife
  B Is unlikely to be successfully reversed when Filshie clips have been used
  C A period of 3 months after the operation is necessary before it can be presumed all ova have been eliminated from the fallopian tubes
  D Causes menorrhagia
  E Has a higher failure rate if the procedure is performed immediately post-partum

B15 **Which of the following clinical symptoms occur with an ectopic pregnancy?:**
  A Vaginal bleeding
  B Amenorrhoea
  C Recurrent abdominal pain
  D Dizziness
  E Shoulder tip pain

B16 **A sperm sample is abnormal if:**
  A The volume is 1 ml^3
  B The sperm concentration is 5 million/ml^3
  C 45% of sperm have forward motility
  D 50% of sperm have normal oval forms
  E There are more than 10 white blood cells (wbc) per high powered field

B17 **Instrumental delivery in a GP unit should not be attempted if:**
  A The cervix is 9 cm dilated
  B The head is not palpable abdominally
  C The membranes are intact
  D The woman has not been catheterised
  E The position of the presenting part has not been determined

B18 **The second stage of labour:**
  A Normally lasts no longer than 1 hour in primigravida, and 30 minutes in multigravida
  B Causes flexion and internal rotation of the head at delivery
  C Should be conducted in the lithotomy position in primigravida
  D Is more likely to end with forceps with an epidural in situ
  E May be heralded by vomiting

B19 **Stress incontinence:**
  A Is more common in nulliparous women
  B Is best treated by terodolin
  C May be prevented by para-urethral pressure during pelvic examination
  D Is unlikely to occur with urge incontinence
  E Has been shown to be prevented by pelvic floor exercises post delivery

B20 **Vulval warts:**
  A Are usually spread by sexual contact
  B Are unaffected by pregnancy
  C Are best treated with podophyllin during pregnancy
  D Are implicated in cancer of the cervix
  E Can be transmitted to a neonate during birth

B21 **An elderly woman with pruritus vulvae presenting to her GP:**
  A Requires a full blood count
  B Should have a urine test for glucose
  C Should be referred for vulval biopsy if leukoplakia is present
  D May have psoriasis
  E Should have a high vaginal swab taken

B22 **Anovulation as a cause of subfertility may be treated in general practice by:**
- **A** Weight gain in women with a low body mass index
- **B** Danazol
- **C** Clomiphene
- **D** Pergonal
- **E** Bromocriptine

B23 **A 19-year-old girl who has never had a period:**
- **A** Requires a vaginal examination
- **B** May be normal
- **C** Requires FSH/LH estimation
- **D** Should have a skull X-ray on presentation
- **E** Should have chromosomal evaluation

B24 **Rhesus iso-immunisation:**
- **A** No longer occurs due to the use of anti-D
- **B** Would be prevented by measuring maternal antibodies
- **C** May occur antenatally in primigravida
- **D** May require intra-uterine blood transfusion for the fetus
- **E** Gets better with each pregnancy

B25 **Pelvic pain in a woman of 35 years may be due to:**
- **A** Ovulation (14 days B4 menses)
- **B** Irritable bowel syndrome
- **C** Ectopic pregnancy
- **D** Endometriosis
- **E** Appendicitis

B26 **Vomiting at 10 weeks of pregnancy may be a symptom of:**
- **A** Hyperemesis gravidarum
- **B** Pyelonephritis
- **C** Torsion of an ovarian cyst
- **D** A degenerating fibroid
- **E** Severe pre-eclampsia

B27 **Uterovaginal prolapse:**
- **A** Is termed procidentia when the cervix lies outside the introitus
- **B** May be asymptomatic
- **C** Is best treated by a ring pessary
- **D** May cause retention of urine
- **E** Is prevented by liberal use of episiotomy at delivery

B28 **As a GP, one of your patients has been treated for a hydatidiform mole. Which of the following advice is correct?:**
- **A** The combined oral contraceptive pill must not be used for 1 year
- **B** Pregnancy should be avoided for 12 months
- **C** After treatment the risk of recurrence is the same as for a non-affected woman
- **D** Congenital abnormalities are commoner in subsequent pregnancies ✗
- **E** Uterine pain in the first 2 weeks following evacuation is unlikely to be significant

B29 **Cytological screening for carcinoma of the cervix:**
- **A** Has not reduced the mortality in the UK ✓
- **B** Can stop at 70 years of age if regular smears have previously been normal
- **C** Detects a large number of minor abnormalities in normal women
- **D** Under the new GP contract, a GP is eligible for the higher payment if 80% of his women patients aged 25–64 years have had a smear within the last $5\frac{1}{2}$ years
- **E** Is best done on day 21 of the menstrual cycle (10 - 20)

B30 **Maternal mortality:**
- **A** Only includes deaths from abortion, pregnancy and labour up to 42 days after delivery ✓
- **B** Occurs at a rate of 1 every 10 000 births in the UK ✓
- **C** Is most commonly due to hypertensive disease ✓
- **D** Due to thromboembolism, is commoner in multiparous women over 35 years of age ✓
- **E** Due to Caesarean section, is 5 times greater in emergency than elective section ✓

→ **B31** **A retroverted uterus:**
- **A** Is usually a normal finding (20%)
- **B** Is a common cause of dyspareunia
- **C** Is likely to become incarcerated during pregnancy
- **D** May be due to endometriosis ✓
- **E** Can be surgically treated by laparoscopic methods

B32 **Karyotype 46XX is compatible with:**
- **A** Turner's syndrome
- **B** Klinefelter's syndrome
- **C** Down's syndrome ✓ Balanced translocation
- **D** Treacher Collins syndrome
- **E** Marfan's syndrome